Drivers, Help Yourself

Against Repetitive Injuries

SERUKIAS ARANOS

iUniverse, Inc.

New York   Bloomington

Drivers, Help Yourself
Against Repetitive Injuries

Copyright © 2010 Serukias Aranos

The information, ideas, and suggestions in this book are not intended as a substitute for professional medical advice. Before following any suggestions contained in this book, you should consult your personal physician. Neither the author nor the publisher shall be liable or responsible for any loss or damage allegedly arising as a consequence of your use or application of any information or suggestions in this book.

iUniverse books may be ordered through booksellers or by contacting:

iUniverse
1663 Liberty Drive
Bloomington, IN 47403
www.iuniverse.com
1-800-Authors (1-800-288-4677)

Because of the dynamic nature of the Internet, any Web addresses or links contained in this book may have changed since publication and may no longer be valid. The views expressed in this work are solely those of the author and do not necessarily reflect the views of the publisher, and the publisher hereby disclaims any responsibility for them.

ISBN: 978-1-4401-9997-4 (pbk)
ISBN: 978-1-4401-9998-1 (ebk)

Printed in the United States of America

iUniverse rev. date: January 21, 2010

I would like to dedicate this booklet to my father, Aranos Teclehaimanot. You are my inspiration, my guide in my life and my hero.
Rest in peace.

I would like to say a big thank you to all my family members who have supported me during the completion of this booklet. I would specially like to thank my mother (Belainesh Seyoum) and my sister (Tsega Aranos) for your belief and your support in me. It means a lot to me.

I would also like to thank all my friends who have helped and supported me during this period. I would particularly like to thank Hani (common) for your support from the beginning; I really appreciate it, mate.

Contents

Introduction

This booklet is designed to help drivers combat the daily aches and pains they experience due to the demands of their occupation. One of the terms used for this problem are repetitive strain injury (RSI). This booklet attempts to solve the physical problems that drivers face each day but do not take the necessary steps to solve until they became unbearable. The lack of knowledge and understanding of the problem and the lack of know-how to solve the problem is thought to be the major factors in perpetuating RSI. Although the government and the powers that be recognize the problem, I am afraid not enough priority is given to this issue. This is the main reason and motivation behind my designing this booklet.

Therefore, this booklet has two main functions. The first function is to educate drivers about RSI, about how their bodies are affected by their occupation, and about the specific soft tissues involved. The second function is an exercise program designed to specifically target the soft tissues affected by the occupation and give the body the balance, flexibility, and strength it needs to complete the daily occupation safely.

This booklet is also designed to be simple to understand and execute, with safety being paramount. It is also designed to be universally flexible so different age groups and fitness levels can use the exercises in this program and still achieve their desired target as well as having the option to progress with increased fitness.

Repetitive Strain Injury

THE PROBLEM

Are you one of the fourteen million people in the UK who suffer from RSI? Did you know that 48 percent of all British drivers suffer from RSI? Some of the most common repetitive strain injuries reported by drivers are low back pain, a stiff neck, and shoulder/upper body discomfort (1).

So, what is RSI?RSI is an umbrella term used to describe a variety of diagnostic conditions characterised by *pain* and *discomfort* that develop gradually in soft tissues. Soft tissues include tendons, ligaments, nerves, and muscles. Work activities which are frequent and repetitive, or work activities with awkward postures, will usually result in RSI. Those affected may be in pain during work or when at home.

One of the main physical factors that cause RSI is *trauma*. This is a condition where a part of the body is injured by repeated overuse. Trauma means that we are causing pain and discomfort to an anatomical feature (in this case, the soft tissues). Trauma weakens and damages these anatomical features (by tearing, breakage, or inflammation) causing RSI. Or trauma can cause the anatomical feature to reinforce itself. Reinforcement can be helpful or harmful.

The body reinforces an anatomical feature to strengthen it so that the feature can deal with the stress it is being put through while working. When your body does this without your knowledge or direction, it is harmful and can lead to an imbalance in an anatomical feature which in turn can cause RSI. But when you reinforce your body appropriately yourself, it can be helpful in preventing RSI.

Therefore, your activities during your working hours (such as driving) cause strain on certain soft tissues of your body. These activities, however minute, build up trauma over time and can lead to a breakdown of soft tissues, causing you injuries, pain, and discomfort. It is important to remember that the level of trauma does not have to be constant. The greater the strain, the more it will accelerate the buildup of trauma. However, even minute trauma, when done long enough, can lead to a total collapse of soft tissue (2) (10).

THE SOLUTION

There are many methods of treating RSI. Some of these are physiotherapy, deep message, chiropractic treatment, yoga, Pilates, and acupuncture. This booklet endorses the use of exercise to treat and/or prevent RSI, mainly by using stretching and strengthening programs to help combat this universal problem. Time and time again, scientists have proven that exercise, specifically flexibility and strength training, can play an important role in the prevention and treatment of RSI (16) (17).

This booklet is an exercise guide/prescription of different methods of stretching and strength training. You can do all of the exercises at home for twenty minutes at a time, three to four days a week, to help overcome the small, niggling, but constant job-related pains and discomforts you are feeling and stabilize your body in the areas you use most.

Repetitive Strain Injury and Drivers

Drivers are susceptible to many repetitive strain injuries. As mentioned before, the most common repetitive stain injuries reported by drivers are lower back pain, a stiff neck, and shoulder/upper body pain. Some of the main contributing factors to RSI for drivers are hard physical work, lifting, a static working posture, and vibration from the vehicle. Continuous pressure on the soft tissues for a long period of time will gradually damage them by tearing, breaking, and inflaming this area, which eventually leads to RSI (3) (6) (7).

LOWER BACK PAIN

When driving, your back is in a static position for a long period of time. Also, your posture and the vibration of the vehicle exert constant pressure on your back (6). This force in turn affects all the soft tissues (muscles, tendons, nerves, and ligaments) in your lower back region. If you are also lifting and carrying items as part of your job, this will add to the pressure on the back.

The main muscle groups involved in lower back pain are the lower back muscles, the abdominals, the gluteus (buttocks), and the hamstrings.

1. Usually, tight hamstring and gluteus (buttocks) muscles have a major effect on your lower back stability. Shortened muscles can affect the alignment of the spine and cause back pain. Therefore, stretching these muscle groups will lengthen the shortened muscles and help relieve back pain (4).

2. Abdominal muscles also have a major effect on lower back pain. Having big belly will negatively affect the alignment of your back bones and help weaken the low back region, which causes pain and discomfort. In contrast, having lean and strong abdominal muscles will give support and stability to the lower back region. It is said that strong abdominal muscles are as crucial as strong back muscles for supporting the lower back and preventing lower back pain (4).

3. The last and most important muscle group is the lower back muscles. The lower back is the centre point where the body pressure is absorbed. Also, the lower back muscles play an important part when bending, lifting objects, sitting, and standing. Constant use of these muscles without leaving enough time for recovery can lead to RSI. Therefore, strengthening and stretching these muscle groups is of utmost importance for the stability of the lower back region.

For these three reasons, I have designed an exercise program to specifically target these muscle groups to help with the stability and strength of the lower back region, making this area strong, stable, flexible, and free of pain.

SHOULDER/UPPER BODY PAIN AND DISCOMFORT

When you are driving, your arms are usually extended to hold the steering wheel and turn the vehicle. Staying in this position for long periods of time, combined with the vibration of the vehicle, exerts constant pressure on your shoulders and upper body region (6) (17). A specific way you hold the steering wheel will affect a specific soft tissue.

The main muscle groups involved are your shoulders, chest, and middle and upper back muscles. Extending your arms for a long time while driving will cause strain to the soft tissues of the shoulders and upper body. Therefore, stretching and strengthening these areas should elevate from pain and discomfort in this region. Also, exercise should help give stability and resistance in these regions to help prevent future RSI. It is with these benefits in mind that I have designed the exercise program.

NECK STIFFNESS

Your neck plays an intricate part when you are driving, and it is put through tremendous pressure, as it has to hold your head in an upright position for a long period of time. Holding the head upright for a long period of time, constantly turning the head while driving, and the vibration of the vehicle can cause RSI of the neck (6). RSI of the neck can cause headaches, eyestrain, and pain through the neck, shoulders, arms, and back. Therefore, a driver's neck health is very important.

Stretching and strengthening the neck muscles should help your neck by giving stability to this area. Having strong and flexible neck muscles will help hold your head steady and give you relief from all the RSI symptoms of pain and discomfort.

However, the exercises for the neck do not have to be included with the rest of this exercise program. The reason for this is that most of these neck exercises can be done almost anytime and anywhere. For example, you can do the neck stretches and strength exercises during your break time or any other time of the day. For this reason, the exercises for the neck are not part of the exercise program and have instead been presented at the end of the exercise program to be performed at a time that suits you best.

The Exercise Program

SAFETY

1. This program is designed for people with RSI and for the prevention of RSI. It is advisable that you consult your doctor and get approval before attempting these exercises if you are unsure.

2. Do not overtax yourself. *Listen to your body.* If pain becomes unbearable or the discomfort is great, stop the exercise or slow down.

3. Make sure you workout on a hard, flat surface (no slippery or uneven surfaces). A mat is recommended. Also, make sure you have enough room for maneuvering safely.

4. Trainers, flat shoes, or bare feet are recommended during the exercises. Shoes with heels are considered dangerous and therefore should not be used.

5. Tracksuits, shorts, and T-shirts are recommended during exercises. Jeans or tight clothing are strongly discouraged.

WARM-UP

The idea behind a warm-up is to get your body ready for a workout. Warming up should not take more than five minutes, and you generally know your body is ready when you start to sweat and your muscles feel warm. There are many methods of warming up your body. Below is a suggestion, but you can be inventive if you wish as long as the target is achieved. It is important to note that a warm-up should be slow and progressive. Breathing is essential. Breathe deeply and in sequence—in through the nose and out through the mouth.

- Start by walking on the spot (for about one minute).
- Progress to jogging on the spot (for about one minute).
- Now do twenty–thirty squats; include the arms.
- Follow it with another twenty–thirty lunges, including the arms.
- Go back to jogging on the spot.
- Once you start to sweat and feel warmed up, go back to walking on the spot for about thirty seconds.

Now your body is ready for the workout.

STRETCHING EXERCISES

Important note --- The "point of stretch" is when you feel some tightness and discomfort in the muscles but NO pain.

1. Sit and reach

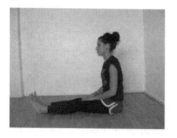 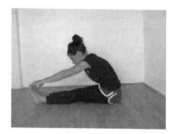

START BY...

- Sitting on the floor with your legs straight out in front of you.

- Keep your legs together, knees pushed into the ground, and toes pointing to the ceiling.

- Now, reach forward with your hands to touch your toes or get as close as you can until you feel the point of stretch.

- Hold this stretch for ten seconds (remember to breathe).

- Relax and slowly get back to the starting position.

- Rest for five seconds.

- Repeat the stretch three times.

- Stand up, shake your legs, and sit back down on the floor.

2.   Hamstring stretch

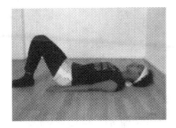 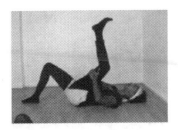

START BY...

- Lying down on your back with your knees slightly bent.

- Raise your left leg and hold it with interlaced fingers on the back of your thigh just under the back of your knee.

- Now, slowly bring your left leg toward your chest as you straighten the knee until you feel the point of stretch.

- Hold for ten seconds (remember to breathe).

- Relax and slowly get back to the starting position.

- Rest for five seconds.

- Now, stretch right leg.

- Repeat the stretch three times for each leg.

- Stand up, shake your legs, and sit back down on the floor.

3.   Piriformis stretch

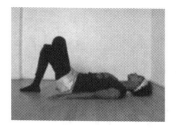 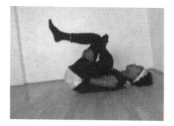

START BY...

- Lying down on the floor with both knees bent.

- Cross your left leg on top of your right leg.

- Raise and hold your legs with interlaced fingers at the back of your right thigh just under the back of your knee.

- Now, pull your knees toward your chest until you feel the point of stretch in your buttocks/hip area.

- Hold for ten seconds (remember to breathe).

- Relax and get back to the starting position.

- Rest for five seconds.

- Now, stretch the other side.

- Repeat the exercise three times for both sides.

- Stand up, shake your legs, and sit back down on the floor.

4.   Hip and lower back stretch

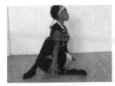 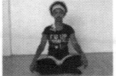 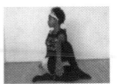

Start by...

- Sitting on the floor with your legs crossed, back straight, and head facing forward.

- Lift and cross your right leg over your left.

- Keep your left leg bent as in the starting position.

- Hug your right leg with your left arm.

- Now, bring your right leg toward your chest as you slowly twist your upper body to look over your right shoulder until you feel the point of stretch in your hip and lower back.

- Hold for ten seconds (remember to breathe).

- Relax and get back to the starting position.

- Rest for five seconds.

- Now, stretch the other side.

- Repeat the exercise three times for both sides.

- Stand up, shake your legs, and sit back down on the floor.

5. Chest stretch

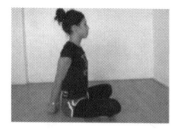 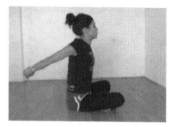

Start by...

- Sitting on the floor with your back straight, legs crossed, and head facing forward (you can also do this exercise sitting in a chair or standing).

- Interlace your fingers behind your back.

- Now, pull both arms up as high as comfortably possible until you feel the point of stretch on your chest area.

- Hold for ten seconds (remember to breathe).

- Relax and slowly return your arms to the starting position.

- Rest for five seconds.

- Repeat this exercise three times.

6.   Reaching stretch

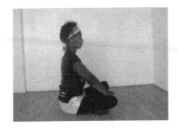 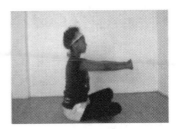

Start by...

- Sitting on the floor with legs crossed, back straight, and head facing forward (you can also do this exercise sitting in a chair or standing).

- Interlace your fingers in front of you with your palms facing away from you.

- Now, slowly straighten your elbows as you raise your arms to shoulder height in front of you until you feel the point of stretch in your upper back, shoulders, and arms.

- Hold for ten seconds (remember to breathe).

- Relax and slowly return your arms to the starting position.

- Rest for five seconds.

- Repeat this exercise three times.

7. Rotation stretch

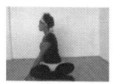 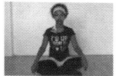 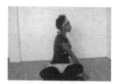

START BY...

- Sitting on the floor with your legs crossed, your back straight, and your head facing forward (you can also do this exercise sitting in a chair or standing).

- Now, slowly turn your upper body to your right as if you are turning to look behind you until you feel the point of stretch your midback area.

- Use your hands to increase the stretch and for balance.

- Hold for ten seconds (remember to breathe).

- Relax and slowly return your upper body to the starting position.

- Rest for five seconds.

- Now, stretch the other side.

- Repeat the exercise three times for each side.

8.   Overhead stretch

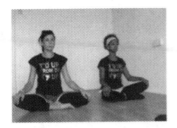 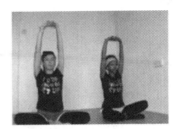

START BY...

- Sitting on the floor with your legs crossed, your back straight, and your head facing forward (you can also do this exercise sitting in a chair or standing).

- Interlace your fingers in front of you.

- Now, slowly straighten your elbows as you raise your arms above your head until you feel the point of stretch.

- Hold for ten seconds (remember to breathe).

- Relax and return your arms to the starting position.

- Repeat the exercise three times.

9.   Shoulder stretch

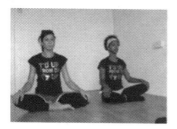 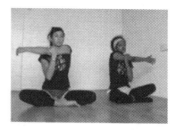

START BY...

- Sitting on the floor with your legs crossed, your back straight, and your head facing forward (you can also do this exercise sitting in a chair or standing).

- Raise your right arm across your body.

- Use your left hand to grab your right arm just above your elbow.

- Your right arm can be straight or bent at the elbow.

- Now, use your left hand to pull your right arm toward your body until you feel the point of stretch in your shoulder.

- Hold for ten seconds (remember to breathe).

- Relax and return to the starting position.

- Now, stretch your right shoulder.

- Repeat this exercise three times.

10. Triceps stretch

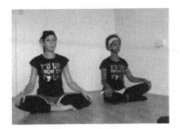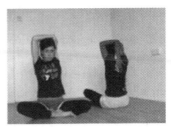

Start by...

- Sitting on the floor with your legs crossed, your back straight, and your head facing forward (you can also do this exercise sitting in a chair or standing).

- Raise both your arms over your head.

- Bend your right elbow and bring your palms down your back.

- Use your left hand to grab your right arm just above your elbow.

- Now, use your left hand to push your right arm slowly toward the middle of your back until you feel the point of stretch in your triceps.

- Hold for ten seconds (remember to breathe).

- Relax and slowly return your arms to the starting position.

- Now, stretch your left arm.

- Repeat this exercise three times.

STRENGTH EXERCISES

The strength exercises are divided into three body parts—the lower back, the neck, and the shoulders and upper body. Choose one of these areas and complete two of the strength exercises. If you can and choose to, you can do more than two exercises. It is important to remember that if you exercise one muscle group, you must also exercise the opposing muscle group in order to achieve balance. For example, if you exercise the abdominal muscles, then you need to exercise the lower back muscles. This same rule applies to the stage of the exercises (beginner, intermediate, and advanced). If you choose a beginner level for the abdominal muscles, then you must choose a beginner level for lower back muscles.

There are many alternative exercises listed for strengthening. The reason is not to confuse you but to give choice so that you may choose the exercise that suits you best. It is recommended that you first choose which part of your body you want to work on (lower back, neck, or shoulders/upper body). You may choose to work on more than one part of your body or all three parts of your body depending on your need. Once you have chosen which part of your body you want/need to strengthen, you can proceed to find your fitness level (beginner, intermediate, or advanced). This can be done by attempting the exercises. Start with a beginner exercise. If you find this easy and not effective, then you may attempt intermediate. It is important to *listen to your body* and not overtax yourself as this may lead to an injury. Once you have found your fitness level, choose from the listed exercises and complete the sets.

ABDOMINAL STRENGTH EXERCISES

BEGINNERS

1. Straight leg raises

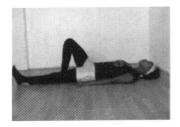 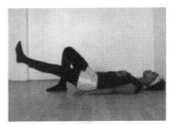

START BY...

- Lying on your back with right leg straight, left leg bent, and left foot flat on the floor.

- Tighten your abdominal muscles to help stabilize your lower back.

- Now, slowly lift your right leg about six to twelve inches off the floor.

- Hold for one second.

- Lower your leg back slowly.

- Attempt to repeat this exercise twelve times for each leg.

- Complete three sets.

2. Mountain climber

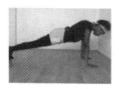 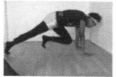 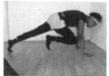

Start by...

- Position yourself in a push-up position.

- Once you get stable, bring your right leg in toward your chest.

- Hold for one second.

- Return to the starting position.

- Now, do the same with your left leg.

- Attempt to repeat this exercise twelve times for each leg.

- Complete three sets.

INTERMEDIATE

1. Half sit-ups

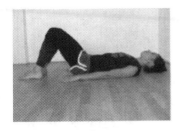 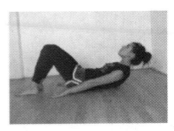

START BY...

- Lying down on your back with knees bent, feet flat on the floor, and arms relaxed by your sides.

- Now, raise your head and shoulder blades off the floor.

- Hold for one second.

- Slowly bring your upper body back to the starting position.

- Attempt to repeat this exercise twelve times.

- Complete three sets.

ADVANCED

1. Full sit-ups

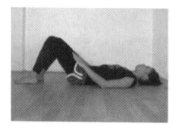 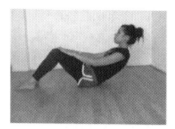

START BY...

-   Lying down on your back with your knees bent and arms resting on your thighs.

-   Now, raise head and shoulders off the floor.

-   Hold for one second.

-   Slowly return your upper body to the starting position.

-   Attempt to repeat this exercise twelve times.

-   Complete three sets.

Lower Back Strength Exercises

Beginner

1. Bird dog

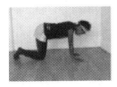 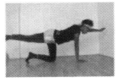 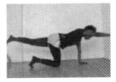

Start by...

- Get on your hands and knees.
- Now, lift and extend your right arm and left leg away from your body.
- Hold for one second.
- Bring your right arm and left leg back to the starting position.
- Relax.
- Now, do the same with your left arm and right leg.
- Attempt to repeat this exercise twelve times for each side.
- Complete three sets.

2. Back leg raise

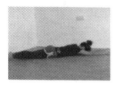 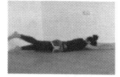 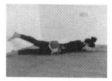

START BY...

- Lying on your stomach with your arms extended out.

- Now, raise your left leg off the ground as high as you can.

- Hold for one second.

- Return your left leg to the starting position.

- Relax.

- Now, do the same with the right leg.

- Attempt to repeat this exercise twelve times.

- Attempt to complete three sets.

3. Back extension

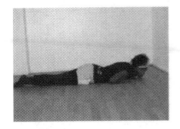 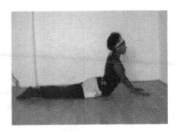

Start by...

- Lying down on your stomach with your arms crossed in front of your head.
- Now, raise your head and chest off the ground using your arms for support.
- Hold for one second.
- Return head and chest back to the starting position.
- Attempt to repeat this exercise twelve times.
- Complete three sets.

INTERMEDIATE

1. Arm and leg back raise

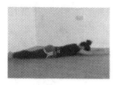 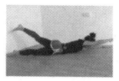 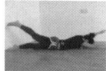

START BY...

- Lying down on your belly with your arms extended out.

- Now, slowly raise your left leg and right arm off the ground as far as you can.

- Hold for one second.

- Return your left leg and right arm slowly back to the starting position.

- Relax.

- Do the same with your right leg and left arm.

- Attempt to repeat this exercise twelve times for each side.

- Complete three sets.

ADVANCED

1.   Back extension

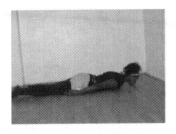 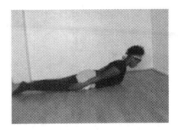

START BY...

- Lying down on your stomach with your arms by the sides of your body.

- Now, slowly raise your head and chest off the ground as far as you can.

- Hold for one second.

- Bring your head and chest slowly back down to the starting position.

- Relax.

- Attempt to repeat this exercise twelve times.

- Complete three sets.

2. Back extension

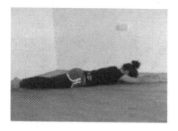 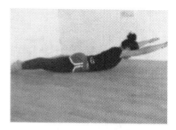

START BY

- Lying down on your stomach with your arms extended out.

- Now, raise your arms, head, and chest off the ground as far as you can.

- Hold for one second.

- Bring your arms, head, and chest back slowly to the starting position.

- Relax.

- Attempt to repeat this exercise twelve times.

- Complete three sets.

Upper Body Strength Exercises

Strength training for the shoulders and upper body is designed slightly different than that for the lower back. For the shoulders and upper body, it is recommended that you choose one or two exercises from the list below.

Beginner

1. Wand exercise

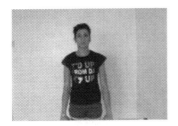 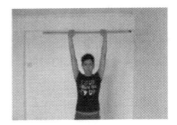

Start by...

- Standing in a stable position with your feet shoulder width apart, knees slightly bent, back straight, and head facing forward

- Get a yardstick or mop handle to use as your wand.

- Grab the wand stick with hands shoulder width apart.

- Now, raise the wand as high overhead as possible.

- Hold for one second.

- Return to the starting position.

- Attempt to repeat this exercise twelve times.

- Complete three sets.

2.   Side arms raise overhead

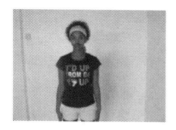 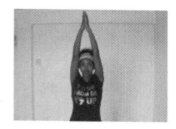

Start by...

- Standing in a stable position with your feet shoulder width apart, knees slightly bent, back straight, and head facing forward.

- Now, raise arms sideways overhead as high as you can, as if you are trying to clap your hands over your head.

- Hold for one second.

- Return to the starting position.

- Attempt to repeat this exercise twelve times.

- Complete three sets.

INTERMEDIATE

1.   Front clap

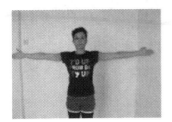 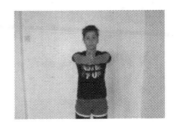

START BY...

-   Standing in a stable position with your feet shoulder width apart, knees slightly bent, back straight, head facing forward, and arms raised away from the body up to shoulder height.

-   Now, bring both arms together as if to clap in front of you.

-   Hold for one second.

-   Return to the starting position.

-   Attempt to repeat this exercise twelve times.

-   Complete three sets.

2. Half press-up

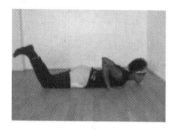 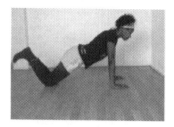

START BY...

- Lying down on your stomach with your hands flat on the floor, shoulder width apart, and your feet raised up off the ground while keeping your knees on the ground.

- Now, raise your body up off the ground without letting your elbows lock.

- Hold for one second.

- Return to the starting position slowly.

- Attempt to repeat this exercise twelve times.

- Complete three sets.

ADVANCED

1. Full press-up

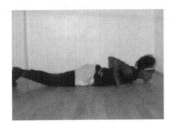 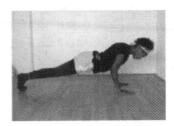

START BY...

- Adopt a position on the floor with your hands shoulder width apart, toes pointed to the floor, and elbows slightly bent (not locked).

- Now, bend your elbows and bring your body down to the ground so that your chest almost touches the ground.

- Hold for one second.

- Now, raise your body back up to the starting position by straitening your elbows but not locking them.

- Hold for one second.

- Attempt to repeat this exercise twelve times.

- Complete three sets.

COOL DOWN

Cool down is very important. Just as a warm-up gets your body ready for work, a cool down completes the exercise. Just like the warm up, the cool down should not take any longer than five minutes. The idea of a cool down is to slowly bring your body from an exercising state to a resting state. It is recommended that everyone complete the exercise with a cool down.

- Start by jogging on the spot (for around three minutes).
- Progress from this by walking on the spot.
- While walking, start to rotate your shoulders.
- Slowly bring down the pace of your walking until you come to a total stop.

The exercise session is now complete.

The Neck Exercise Program

When exercising the neck, there are limited movements available to us because of the mobility and the sensitivity of the neck area. Therefore, the following program will deal with four different movements—neck flexion, neck extension, neck rotation, and neck side bend. These movements will be used for warm up, stretching, and strength exercises.

WARM-UP AND STRENGTHENING NECK EXERCISES

1. Neck extension

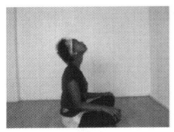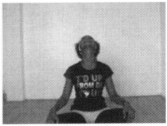

START BY...

- Sitting on the floor with your back straight, legs crossed, head facing forward, and arms resting on your legs.

- Now, slowly tilt your head back as far as you can so that your chin is pointing towards the ceiling.

- Hold for one second.

- Relax and bring your head back to the starting position.

- Attempt to repeat this exercise twelve times.

- Complete three sets.

2. Neck flexion

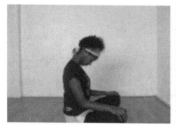 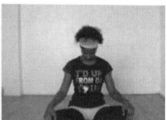

Start by...

- Sitting on the floor with your back straight, legs crossed, head facing forward, and arms resting on your legs.

- Now, slowly bend your head forward and down, allowing your chin to drop towards your chest as far as you can.

- Hold for one second.

- Relax and return your head back to the starting position.

- Attempt to repeat this exercise twelve times.

- Complete three sets.

3. Neck rotation

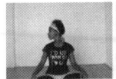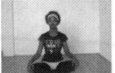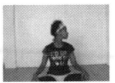

START BY...

- Sitting on the floor with your back straight, legs crossed, head facing forward, and arms resting on your legs.

- Now, slowly turn your head to one side as though you are trying to look over your shoulder as far as you can.

- Hold for one second.

- Relax and return your head back to the starting position.

- Attempt to repeat this exercise twelve times.

- Complete three sets.

- Now, do the same exercise for the opposing side.

4. Neck side bends

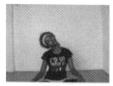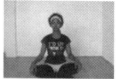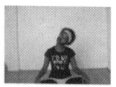

Start by...

- Sitting on the floor with your back straight, legs crossed, head facing forward, and arms resting on your legs.

- Now, slowly tilt your head to one side, moving your ears toward your shoulder as far as you can.

- Hold for one second.

- Relax and return your head to the starting position.

- Attempt to repeat this exercise twelve times for each side.

- Complete three sets.

Now you are ready to stretch your neck.

NECK STRETCHES

1. Neck extension

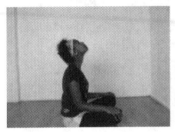 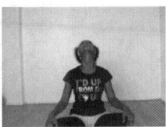

START BY...

- Sitting on the floor with your back straight, legs crossed, head facing forward, and arms resting on your legs.

- Now, slowly tilt your head back so that your chin is pointing towards the ceiling until you feel the point of stretch.

- Hold for ten seconds (remember to breathe).

- Relax and bring your head back to the starting position.

- Repeat this exercise three times.

2. Neck flexion

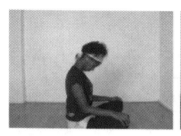 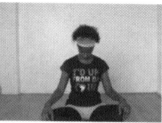

Start by...

-   Sitting on the floor with your back straight, legs crossed, head facing forward, and arms resting on your legs.

-   Now, slowly bend your head forward and down, allowing your chin to drop towards your chest until you feel the point of stretch.

-   Hold for ten seconds (remember to breathe).

-   Relax and return your head back to the starting position.

-   Repeat this exercise three times.

3.   Neck rotation

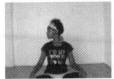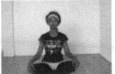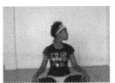

START BY...

- Sitting on the floor with your back straight, legs crossed, head facing forward, and arms resting on your legs.

- Now, slowly turn your head to one side as though you are trying to look over your shoulder until you feel the point of stretch.

- Hold for ten seconds (remember to breathe).

- Relax and return your head back to the starting position.

- Now, stretch the other side.

- Repeat exercise three times for both sides.

4.   Neck side bends

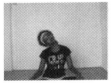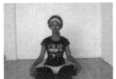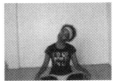

START BY...

- Sitting on the floor with your back straight, legs crossed, head facing forward, and arms resting on your legs.

- Now, slowly tilt your head to one side, moving your ears toward your shoulder until you feel the point of stretch.

- Hold for ten seconds (remember to breathe).

- Relax and return your head to the starting position.

- Now, stretch the other side.

- Repeat this exercise three times for each side.

Neck exercise is now complete.

Conclusion

It is the sincere hope that this exercise program works for you and that you have a better understanding of how your body is affected by your occupation. Some important things to remember are that your body is unique. Therefore, it is essential that you listen to your body and work with it. Take your time and progress slowly. If at anytime you feel that something does not feel right, I suggest you stop and consult your doctor.

'What you reap is what you sow'. How much dedication you put into this will determined what you get out of it. This does not mean that you should overdo this. Do not do this exercise more than once a day; give your body the time to recover. If you have any queries about any of the issues raised in this booklet I can be contacted at helpyourselfdrivers@ hotmail.co.uk.

References

1. Motortorque.com. repetitive Driving Injuries – How Do You Rate? file://localhost/E:/Repetitive%20Driving%20 Injuries%20-%20statistics_.mht
2. About.com:Ergonomics. Do you suffer from repetitive driving injuries? http://ergonomics.about.com/od/every-dayergonomics/qt/repdriveinjury.htm
3. Occupational Health Clinics for Ontario Workers Inc. Ergonomics and Driving: Is Driving really bad for you? http://www.ohcow.on.ca/resources/handbooks/ergonomics_driving/Ergonomics_And_Driving.htm
4. bigbackpain.com. Exercise to help prevent back pain. http://www.bigbackpain.com/back_exercises.html
5. bbchealth.co.uk/health. Back pain. http://www.bbc.co.uk/health/conditions/back_pain/index.shtml
6. Mansfield, N J; Marshall, J M. symptoms of musculoskeletal disorders in stages rally drivers and co-drivers. British Journal of Sports Medicine: Volume 35(5) October 2001pp 314-320.
7. Canadian Driver. Drivers at risk from repetitive strain injuries. February 27, 2008. http://www.canadiandriver.com/
8. Gear Up "lose the crank!". Upper Extremity Injuries in the Trucking Industry. http://gearuplosethecrank.com/gear_up_trucker_injuries.html

9. Robert J. Daul, MPT. Easy Exercise Program for Low Back Pain Relief. Spine-health, Trusted Information for pain Relief. http://www.spine-health.com/wellness/exercise/easy-exercise-program-low-back-pain-relief

10. CCOHS. Work-related Musculoskeletal Disorders (WMSDs). http://www.ccohs.ca/oshanswers/diseases/rmirsi.html

11. Osteopathclinic.com. Exercise for the Lumber (Lower Back) Region. http://www.osteopathclinic.com/exercises/lumbar.html

12. The Physiotherapy Site. Simple Neck Exercises. http://www.thephysiotherapysite.co.uk/physiotherapy/exercise/simple-neck-exercises

13. The Chartered Society of Physiotherapy. Repetitive strain injury (RSI) still blights British workers. http://www.csp.org.uk/director/press/pressreleases.cfm?item_id=94919D04DEF6F9D2538544B581A5DF50

14. About.com:Ergonomics. What causes Repetitive Strain Injuries? http://ergonomics.about.com/od/repetitivestressinjuries/a/rsicauses.htm

15. AAOS. Low Back Exercise Guide. http://orthoinfo.aaos.org/topic.cfm?topic=A00302

16. RSI – vereniging. RSI Treatment. http://www.rsi-vereniging.nl/index.php?option=com_content&task=view&id=101&Itemid=107

17. Verhagen A, Karels C, Bierma-Zeinstra S, Feleus A, Dahaghin S, Burdorf A, Koes B. Exercise proves effective in a systematic review of work-related complaints of the arm, neck, or shoulder. Journal of Clinical Epidemiology. Volume 60, Issue 2, pages 110.e1-110.e14.